PELVIC PAIN CURE

An essential guidebook on how to treat pelvic pain effectively

Dr Rowan Theo

Table of Contents

CHAPTER ONE

What is Pelvic Pain?

o Pelvic ache in particular happens in the vicinity of the decrease stomach. The ache may be regular or come and go. It may be a sharp, stabbing ache in a particular region or a stupid pain that spreads. If the ache is excessive, it may intrude together along with your each day activities.

o If you're a lady, you can enjoy ache all through your length. It also can show up if you have intercourse. Pelvic ache may be a signal of a hassle with an organ on your pelvic region, inclusive of the uterus, ovaries, fallopian tubes, cervix, or vagina. If you're male, the reason can be a prostate hassle. In each guys and ladies, it may be a symptom of contamination or a hassle with the urinary tract, decrease intestines, rectum, muscle tissues, or bones. Some ladies have a couple of reason of pelvic ache simultaneously.

Causes:

• The maximum common reasons of pelvic ache in guys:

Urinary tract contamination (UTI):

• A urinary tract contamination is a bacterial contamination someplace alongside the urinary tract that consists of the urethra, bladder, ureters, and kidneys. UTIs are a common complaint, and a greater common symptom is ache in the decrease stomach or pelvis.

• **Other signs and symptoms consist of:**

o A burning sensation while urinating

o Need to urinate regularly

o Changes in the colour or smell of urine

o Fever or chills

o Pain in different regions, like facets or decrease again

Sexually transmitted contamination (STI):

o Some STIs, like gonorrhea and chlamydia, additionally reason pelvic ache. The Centers for Disease Control and Prevention (CDC) estimates that 2.86 million chlamydia infections arise in the United States every year.

o Symptoms consist of:

Pain in the pelvis

Inflammation of the urethra

 Discharge from the penis

o Chlamydia also can infect the rectum or anus, probably inflicting ache there as nicely.

o A circumstance referred to as lymphogranuloma venereal can end result from specific variations of the micro organism that reason chlamydia. This can result in pelvic ache this is hard to deal with.

o   The   CDC   notes   that lymphogranuloma   venereum   can reason outbreaks of proctitis, or irritation of the anus and rectum, in guys who've intercourse with guys.

o The contamination can reason signs and symptoms inclusive of ache and discharge from the penis. If it impacts the rectum, it may reason a discharge from the anus or painful stools.

Prostatitis:

o Prostatitis is an irritation of the prostate, a tiny gland in the male reproductive device. The prostate produces fluid, which enters the semen.

• There are some forms of prostatitis:

• Acute bacterial prostatitis:

o This circumstance effects from a bacterial contamination of the prostate. Bacteria can attain the gland thru the urethra, and as they spread, they could reason ache in the pelvis, groin, or decrease again.

o Acute bacterial prostatitis also can reason pain in the penis or testicles. Pain can also additionally accompany different signs and symptoms, inclusive of:

A burning sensation all through urination

Fever

Chills

Nausea and vomiting

Difficulty urinating

Frequent urination

Urinary blockage or lack of ability to urinate

A susceptible or damaged urine stream

Waking up regularly at night time to urinate

 Painful ejaculation

o A bacterial contamination of the prostate may be critical and absolutely everyone with those signs and symptoms need to see a health practitioner right now. A urologist can deal with a bacterial contamination with antibiotics.

CHAPTER TWO

Chronic bacterial prostatitis:

o Chronic bacterial prostatitis is a common contamination in the prostate. Symptoms are like the ones of acute bacterial prostatitis, despite the fact that they'll be much less excessive.

o A urologist will normally deal with it with a low dose of antibiotics, or a mixture of antibiotics, over an extended length.

o If the hassle is inflicting trouble passing urine, the urologist can also additionally prescribe medicines referred to as alpha-blockers to assist loosen up the bladder and surrounding muscle tissues so the frame can launch urine.

• **Non-bacterial prostatitis**:

• Long-lasting irritation of the prostate can end result from non-bacterial prostatitis, a sort of persistent pelvic ache syndrome. Doctors aren't certain of the precise reason of this circumstance. It's crucial to recognize that the irritation has not anything to do with a bacterial contamination, so it might not reply nicely to antibiotics.

•   Asymptomatic inflammatory prostatitis:

• Prostatitis can reason certainly no signs and symptoms. Blood assessments can also additionally display a better wide variety of white blood cells, and docs will need to rule out prostate most cancers earlier than creating a diagnosis.

Hernia:

o Sudden decrease belly ache can imply a hernia.

o A hernia develops while a chunk of tissue or gut pushes thru a weakness in the muscle tissues. It regularly bureaucracy a small painful swelling in the vicinity.

o The ache can also additionally worsen while the man or woman places a pressure at the muscle tissues, inclusive of laughing, coughing, or lifting.

Irritable Bowel Syndrome (IBS):

- IBS generally reasons signs and symptoms alongside the intestinal tract, inclusive of:

o Painful cramps

o Bloating

o Diarrhea

o Constipation

o Mucus in stool

- These signs and symptoms normally disappear briefly after stool.

Appendicitis:

• The appendix is a small organ at the proper facet of the frame, and irritation of the appendix can reason pelvic ache.

• **Other signs and symptoms consist of:**

o Fever

o Loss of appetite

o Nausea and vomiting

o Swelling of the decrease stomach

• If sharp ache in the decrease proper stomach accompanies any of the above signs and symptoms, are looking for clinical interest right now. Surgery can be necessary.

CHAPTER THREE

Urinary Stones:

o Urinary stones are shaped while salts or minerals, inclusive of calcium, increase in the urine and the frame has trouble casting off them. These minerals can clump collectively and crystallize in urinary stones.

o Stones have a tendency to reason signs and symptoms best while the frame attempts to by skip them, and ache in the pelvis or decrease again is common. Other adjustments consist of trouble passing urine and blood in the urine.

o Doctors can also additionally prescribe ache relievers to assist by skip the stones, and a few medicines can split the stones. Larger stones require surgical operation in a few cases.

Cystitis:

o Cystitis is irritation of the bladder, normally as a consequence of contamination.

o It reasons ache in the pelvis, observed via way of means of signs and symptoms inclusive of:

o Difficulty urinating

o Poor urine output

o Having to urinate regularly

o Burning ache while urinating

o Blood in urine

o Changes in the advent or smell of urine

• A health practitioner will normally use a quick route of antibiotics to deal with a bladder contamination.

Urethral Stenosis:

• Urethral stricture happens while the urethra shrinks or blockages, making it hard for the urine to flow. In addition to decrease belly ache, signs and symptoms consist of:

o Pain while urinating

o Difficulty urinating

o Urine leak

o Blood or urine performing in semen

o Loss of bladder control

• Treatment entails surgical operation, and those vary.

Benign Prostatic Hyperplasia (BPH):

• BPH happens while the prostate receives larger because of some thing apart from most cancers. As the prostate enlarges, it places stress at the urethra. This can reason trouble passing urine and ache in the pelvis. Eventually, the muscle tissues of the bladder can also additionally weaken from the tension, which makes signs and symptoms worse.

• The maximum common reasons of pelvic ache in Women:

Menstrual Pain and Cramps:

o Menstrual ache and cramps are a common reason of pelvic ache in ladies.

o More than 1/2 of ladies who've their length will enjoy ache for as a minimum 1 to two days in every cycle.

o Period cramps normally arise right now earlier than a lady begins off evolved her length due to the fact the uterus contracts and loses its lining. The ache can also additionally seem like a muscle spasm or a stinging ache.

o Using a heat heating pad can ease the sensation. Over-the-counter medicines, inclusive of ibuprofen (Advil) and naproxen (Aleve), also can assist relieve ache.

o In case of excessive ache because of menstruation, docs can also additionally suggest different medicines.

CHAPTER FOUR

Ovulation:

o When a lady ovulates, the ovaries launch an egg and different fluids. The egg will then journey thru the fallopian tube and into the uterus. Fluid launched via way of means of the ovary can journey to the pelvic vicinity, on occasion inflicting pelvic infection and ache.

o The pain can ultimate for mins or hours and extrade facets of the frame, relying on which ovary launched the egg. The ache is brief and does now no longer require any unique remedy.

Interstitial cystitis:

o It is likewise feasible that a lady suffers from endured irritation of the bladder without a acknowledged reason. The clinical time period for that is interstitial cystitis, and docs presently do not know why this takes place.

o Interstitial cystitis can reason pelvic ache and signs and symptoms inclusive of painful urination, the want to urinate regularly, and ache all through intercourse. Treatment regularly entails handling the signs and symptoms in addition to feasible.

Cystitis:

o Cystitis refers to irritation of the bladder because of a bacterial contamination. This takes place due to the fact micro organism from the vagina, rectum, or pores and skin can input the urethra and journey to the bladder.

o A urinary tract contamination (UTI) can arise everywhere in the device, even as cystitis best happens in the bladder.

o Both situations are common in ladies. Sometimes those infections will depart on their own, however a quick route of antibiotics will normally deal with cystitis and different UTIs.

Sexually Transmitted Infections:

o Pelvic ache can also additionally imply the presence of a sexually transmitted contamination (STI) inclusive of gonorrhea or chlamydia. STIs arise in sexually lively human beings.

o In addition to pelvic ache, different signs and symptoms of STIs can consist of painful urination, bleeding among periods, and adjustments in vaginal discharge.

o Anyone who studies those adjustments need to see their health practitioner who may be capable of diagnose an STI and prescribe remedy, normally inclusive of antibiotics. It is likewise important to allow sexual companions understand approximately the contamination to save you it from spreading.

Pelvic Inflammatory Disease:

o Pelvic inflammatory disease (PID) is an contamination of the uterus that may harm surrounding tissue. PID can arise if micro organism from the vagina or cervix input the uterus and settle.

o It is mostly a trouble of an STI inclusive of gonorrhea or chlamydia. In addition to pelvic ache, ladies can also additionally enjoy different signs and symptoms, inclusive of unusual vaginal discharge and bleeding.

o IRS will increase the chance of infertility in ladies. The CDC notes that 1 in eight ladies who've had PID additionally have problem getting pregnant.

o Treatment normally entails taking antibiotics to deal with the bacterial contamination. However, they can not deal with scars, that is why early remedy is crucial.

Endometriosis:

o Endometriosis happens while the endometrium, or tissue that traces the internal of the uterus, grows outdoor the uterus.

o Endometriosis may be a supply of persistent and lasting pelvic ache in a few ladies. When a man or woman's length starts off evolved, this tissue outdoor the uterus responds to hormonal adjustments, that can reason bleeding and irritation in the pelvis.

o Some human beings can also additionally enjoy slight to excessive ache. Endometriosis could make it hard for a few ladies to get pregnant. Doctors can also additionally suggest a lot of remedies, relying at the severity of the signs and symptoms.

Irritable bowel syndrome (IBS):

o Irritable Bowel Syndrome (IBS) is an intestinal sickness that reasons ache and signs and symptoms, inclusive of constipation, diarrhea, and bloating.

o Symptoms of IBS have a tendency to flare up and depart over time, particularly after a bowel movement. There isn't any therapy for IBS, so remedy specializes in handling signs and symptoms thru adjustments in diet, pressure levels, and medicines.

CHAPTER FIVE

Appendicitis:

o Appendicitis is irritation of the appendix, that is a small organ placed in the decrease proper stomach. This circumstance is because of contamination, and even though it is common, it may be critical.

o Anyone experiencing sharp ache in the decrease proper stomach, in conjunction with different signs and symptoms inclusive of vomiting and fever, need to see a health practitioner right now, as this will be a signal of appendicitis.

Urinary stones:

o Stones in the urinary tract are made from salts and minerals, inclusive of calcium, which the frame has trouble in passing thru urine.

o These minerals can increase and shape crystals in the bladder or kidneys which regularly reason ache in the pelvis or decrease again. Stones also can reason urine to extrade colour, regularly turning it crimson or reddish with blood.

o Some stones do now no longer require remedy, however passing them may be painful. At different times, a health practitioner can also additionally suggest medication to interrupt up the stones or surgical operation to dispose of them.

Ectopic being pregnant:

o An ectopic being pregnant happens while an embryo implants everywhere outdoor the uterus and starts off evolved to develop.

o A lady can also additionally enjoy very sharp ache and cramp in her pelvis, that is normally focused on one facet. Other signs and symptoms consist of nausea, vaginal bleeding, and dizziness.

o Anyone who suspects an ectopic being pregnant need to see a health practitioner right now, as it's miles a probably deadly circumstance.

Pelvic adhesions

o An adhesion is scar tissue that happens in the frame and connects problems that need to now no longer be connected. This can result in ache, because the frame has a difficult time adjusting to the grip.

o Scar tissue can shape because of an vintage contamination, endometriosis, or different troubles in the vicinity. Pelvic adhesions can result in persistent pelvic ache in a few ladies, and they could reason different signs and symptoms, relying on in which the scar tissue appears.

o A health practitioner can also additionally suggest minimally invasive surgical procedures to assist lessen adhesions and relieve signs and symptoms.

Ovarian cysts:

o Ovarian cysts arise while the ovaries fail to launch an egg. The follicle containing the egg won't absolutely open to launch the egg, or it can be clogged with fluid.

o When this takes place, a boom referred to as cyst bureaucracy in the vicinity, that can reason bloating, stress, or pelvic ache at the facet of the frame with the cyst.

o In many cases, ovarian cysts depart on their own. In a few cases, a cyst can bleed or burst, that can reason excessive, excessive ache in the pelvis and can require clinical remedy.

o Doctors can pick out ovarian cysts the usage of ultrasound, and they could suggest remedies starting from watchful ready to surgical operation.

Uterine fibroids:

o Fibroids are portions of muscle and fibrous tissue in the uterus. Although they're now no longer cancerous and do now no longer have a tendency to reason signs and symptoms, those growths may be a supply of ache. They can reason pain in the pelvis or decrease again or ache all through intercourse.

o   Fibroids also can reason immoderate bleeding or cramping all through menstruation.

o Some fibroids do now no longer require remedy. If a lady reveals her signs and symptoms hard to manage, docs can also additionally suggest one of the many remedies, inclusive of medicines, non-invasive procedures, or surgical operation.

CHAPTER SIX

Tumor:

o In uncommon cases, malignant boom of the reproductive device, urinary tract, or gastrointestinal device may be the reason of pelvic ache. The tumor also can reason different signs and symptoms, relying on in which it appears.

o Doctors will want to do a radical evaluation, regularly the usage of blood assessments and imaging, to pick out a tumor. Once they diagnose the hassle, they'll suggest feasible remedies.

Diagnosis:

• Determining what's inflicting your persistent pelvic ache regularly entails a technique of elimination, as many issues can reason pelvic ache.

• In addition to an in depth interview approximately your ache, non-public clinical history, and own circle of relatives history, your health practitioner can also additionally ask you to hold a diary of your ache and different signs and symptoms.

• Tests or assessments your health practitioner would possibly propose consist of:

• Pelvic exam: This can also additionally display symptoms and symptoms of contamination, unusual growths, or tight pelvic ground muscle tissues. Your health practitioner exams for regions of tenderness. Tell your health practitioner in case you enjoy any pain all through this check, particularly if the ache is much like the ache you felt.

• Lab assessments: During the pelvic exam, your health practitioner can also additionally ask labs to test for infections, inclusive of chlamydia or gonorrhea. Your health practitioner may additionally order blood assessments to test your blood depend and a urinalysis to search for a urinary tract contamination.

• Ultrasound: This check makes use of high-frequency sound waves to supply unique pix of the systems on your frame. This process is particularly beneficial for locating lumps or cysts in the ovaries, uterus, or fallopian tubes.

• Other imaging assessments: Your health practitioner can also additionally suggest belly x-rays, computed tomography (CT), or magnetic resonance imaging (MRI) to assist discover unusual systems or growths.

• Laparoscopy: During this surgical operation, your health practitioner makes a small incision on your stomach and inserts a skinny tube connected to a small camera (laparoscope). The laparoscope lets in your health practitioner to view your pelvic organs and search for abnormal tissue or symptoms and symptoms of contamination: this process is particularly beneficial for detecting endometriosis and persistent pelvic inflammatory disease.

• Finding the underlying reason of persistent pelvic ache may be an extended technique, and on occasion a easy rationalization can also additionally in no way be found.

Treatment:

• Treatment for pelvic ache varies relying at the reason, the depth of the ache, and the way regularly the ache happens. Sometimes pelvic ache is dealt with medicine, inclusive of antibiotics. If the ache effects from a hassle with any of the pelvic organs, remedy can also additionally contain surgical operation or different procedures. Physiotherapy can on occasion be beneficial. Plus, given that dwelling with persistent pelvic ache may be demanding and overwhelming, research have proven the advantage of operating with a educated counselor, psychologist, or psychiatrist maximum of the time. A health practitioner can offer greater statistics approximately the specific remedies for pelvic ache.

When to go to a Doctor?

• Temporary, slight pelvic ache might be not anything to fear approximately. If the ache is excessive or persists for greater than a week, make an appointment together along with your health practitioner.

• You need to see the medical doctor in case you enjoy:

o Blood in urine

o Foul-smelling urine

o Difficulty urinating

o Inability to have a bowel movement

o Bleeding among periods

o Fever

o Chills

Home Remedies:

• Pelvic ache regularly responds to over the counter ache relievers, however make sure to seek advice from your health practitioner earlier than taking any sort of medicine all through being pregnant.

• In a few cases, relaxation can assist. In others, mild actions and mild exercising may be greater beneficial. Try those tips:

o Place a warm water bottle for your stomach to peer if it facilitates relieve the cramps or take a heat bath.

o Elevate your legs. This can assist relieve pelvic ache and ache, which impacts the decrease again or thighs.

o Try yoga, prenatal yoga, and meditation, which also can be beneficial for ache management.

o Take herbs, inclusive of willow bark, that can assist lessen ache.

Obtain your health practitioner's approval earlier than the usage of it all through being pregnant.

THE END